Hyper Ketosis Diet

A Beginner's 5-Step Quick Start Guide for Women, with Sample Recipes and a Meal Plan

copyright © 2024 Mary Golanna

All rights reserved No part of this book may be reproduced, or stored in a retrieval system, or transmitted in any form or by any means, electronic, mechanical, photocopying, recording, or otherwise, without express written permission of the publisher.

Disclaimer

By reading this disclaimer, you are accepting the terms of the disclaimer in full. If you disagree with this disclaimer, please do not read the guide.

All of the content within this guide is provided for informational and educational purposes only, and should not be accepted as independent medical or other professional advice. The author is not a doctor, physician, nurse, mental health provider, or registered nutritionist/dietician. Therefore, using and reading this guide does not establish any form of a physician-patient relationship.

Always consult with a physician or another qualified health provider with any issues or questions you might have regarding any sort of medical condition. Do not ever disregard any qualified professional medical advice or delay seeking that advice because of anything you have read in this guide. The information in this guide is not intended to be any sort of medical advice and should not be used in lieu of any medical advice by a licensed and qualified medical professional.

The information in this guide has been compiled from a variety of known sources. However, the author cannot attest to or guarantee the accuracy of each source and thus should not be held liable for any errors or omissions.

You acknowledge that the publisher of this guide will not be held liable for any loss or damage of any kind incurred as a result of this guide or the reliance on any information provided within this guide. You acknowledge and agree that you assume all risk and responsibility for any action you undertake in response to the information in this guide.

Using this guide does not guarantee any particular result (e.g., weight loss or a cure). By reading this guide, you acknowledge that there are no guarantees to any specific outcome or results you can expect.

All product names, diet plans, or names used in this guide are for identification purposes only and are the property of their respective owners. The use of these names does not imply endorsement. All other trademarks cited herein are the property of their respective owners.

Where applicable, this guide is not intended to be a substitute for the original work of this diet plan and is, at most, a supplement to the original work for this diet plan and never a direct substitute. This guide is a personal expression of the facts of that diet plan.

Where applicable, persons shown in the cover images are stock photography models and the publisher has obtained the rights to use the images through license agreements with third-party stock image companies.

Table of Contents

Introduction	7
Understanding Hyper Ketosis for Women	9
How Does Hyper Ketosis Diet Work?	10
Use Cases of Hyper Ketosis Diet	12
Principles of the Hyper Ketosis Diet	14
Disadvantages of the Hyper Ketosis Diet	20
Potential Side Effects of the Hyper Ketosis Diet	21
5-Step Plan to Get Started with the Hyper Ketosis Diet for Women	23
Step 1: Educate Yourself About the Hyper Ketosis Diet	23
Step 2: Clean Out Your Pantry	25
Step 3: Plan Your Meals	29
Step 4: Track Your Progress	34
Benefits of Monitoring Progress	37
Importance of Regular Review	38
Step 5: Stay Motivated and Adjust as Needed	38
Tips for Success	41
Foods to Eat	42
Foods to Avoid	43
7-Day Sample Meal Plan	45
Sample Recipes	48
Keto-Friendly Pancakes	49
Chicken Caesar Wrap	51
Beef Fajita Bowl	53
Ham and Cheese Omelet with Sautéed Mushrooms	55
Tofu and Vegetable Stir-Fry	57
Baked Cod	60
Avocado Toast with Smoked Salmon on Low-Carb Bread	63
Caesar Salad with Grilled Chicken Breast	65

Spaghetti Squash Bolognese	67
Keto-Friendly Granola with Almond Milk	70
Zucchini Noodles with Shrimp Scampi	72
Grilled Pork Chops with Asparagus and Garlic Butter Sauce	74
Turkey and Cheese Roll-Ups with Cucumber Slices	76
Baked Chicken Thighs	78
Tuna Salad Wrap	80
Beef Stir-Fry with Vegetables over Zucchini Noodles	82
Spinach and Feta Omelet with Avocado Slices	85
Grilled Chicken Salad	87
Baked Salmon with Broccoli and Cauliflower Rice	89
Conclusion	**91**
FAQs	**94**
References and Helpful Links	**97**

Introduction

Enhancing your health and vitality often starts with making well-informed dietary choices. The Hyper Ketosis Diet is a tailored nutritional strategy that provides a distinctive method for women's wellness, concentrating on energy balance, enhancing mental sharpness, and aiding in weight control.

Hyper ketosis goes beyond simply cutting carbs. It involves adopting a lifestyle that helps you tap into your body's natural energy reserves. By emphasizing high-fat, low-carb meals, this diet propels your body into a heightened state of ketosis, where fat becomes the primary source of fuel. This metabolic shift can lead to increased energy, sharper mental clarity, and effective weight management.

Women encounter unique health challenges, including hormonal fluctuations and varying metabolic rates. The Hyper Ketosis Diet addresses these differences by helping stabilize insulin levels, reduce inflammation, and support hormonal balance. It is particularly beneficial for managing conditions like polycystic ovary syndrome (PCOS) or insulin resistance.

In this guide, we will talk about the following;

- Understanding Hyper Ketosis
- How Does Hyper Ketosis Work?
- Use Cases of Hyper Ketosis Diet
- Benefits and Potential Disadvantages of The Hyper Ketosis Diet
- Potential Side Effects
- 5-Step Plan to Getting Started with Hyper Ketosis Diet
- Foods to Eat and To Avoid
- Sample Meal Plan and Sample Recipes

Keep reading to discover more about the specific benefits of Hyper ketosis for women. By the end of this guide, you will have a firm understanding of how this dietary plan can optimize your well-being and empower you to thrive in all aspects of life. So, let's delve deeper into the world of Hyper ketosis and discover its transformative effects for women.

Understanding Hyper Ketosis for Women

Ketosis is a metabolic condition in which your body transitions from relying on carbohydrates for energy to using fats. This change happens when you drastically cut down on carbohydrate consumption, causing the liver to transform stored fat into ketones. These ketones act as an alternative energy source for both the body and brain, offering several health advantages.

The Hyper Ketosis diet emphasizes a specific macronutrient distribution: high fat, moderate protein, and low carbohydrates. Typically, your daily intake should consist of about 70-75% fats, 20-25% proteins, and only 5-10% carbohydrates. This balance encourages the body to enter and maintain ketosis, optimizing fat-burning and energy levels.

For women, ketosis can offer unique benefits and challenges. The diet may help balance hormones, improve insulin sensitivity, and support weight management. However, women may experience different metabolic responses due to hormonal fluctuations, especially related to menstrual cycles.

Understanding these nuances can help tailor the diet to better suit female physiology, ensuring both effectiveness and sustainability.

How Does Hyper Ketosis Diet Work?

The Hyper Ketosis Diet works by pushing the body into a state of hyper ketosis, which is an intensified version of ketosis. Here's how it functions in the body:

1. *Carbohydrate Restriction*: By drastically cutting carbohydrate consumption to around 20-50 grams daily, the body loses its primary energy source, glucose, commonly obtained from carbohydrates. This limitation compels the body to find other energy sources, triggering a metabolic change.

2. *Increased Fat Intake*: The diet emphasizes high-fat consumption, often comprising 70-80% of daily caloric intake. This high-fat intake becomes the primary energy source for the body. As carbs are limited, this shift encourages the liver to convert stored fats into ketones, which serve as a more stable energy source for the body.

3. *Elevated Ketone Levels*: In hyper ketosis, ketone levels can rise significantly, often exceeding typical ketogenic levels, which are generally around 0.5-3.0 mmol/L. These elevated ketones are used as an

alternative energy source, especially for the brain and muscles, which helps improve focus and stamina during physical activities.

4. *Metabolic Adaptation*: Over time, generally within a few weeks, the body undergoes metabolic adaptation, becoming more efficient at burning fat and utilizing ketones for energy. This adaptation not only aids in weight management but can also enhance physical endurance and mental performance, making it easier for individuals to maintain their energy levels throughout the day.

5. *Potential Benefits*: This state of hyper ketosis may lead to a variety of potential benefits, including improved energy levels, heightened mental clarity, and enhanced metabolic health. Additionally, individuals may experience weight loss, reduced inflammation, and better control of blood sugar levels, making this approach appealing to those seeking to improve overall health and well-being.

The diet requires careful monitoring and adjustment of macronutrient ratios to maintain the hyper ketotic state effectively.

Use Cases of Hyper Ketosis Diet

The Hyper Ketosis diet is not just a popular trend; it offers various practical applications for women looking to improve their health and lifestyle. Here are some specific use cases where this diet can be particularly beneficial:

1. **Weight Loss and Body Composition**
   - *Targeting Stubborn Fat*: Women often struggle with losing fat in areas like hips, thighs, and abdomen. Hyper Ketosis accelerates fat loss by forcing the body to use fat stores for energy.
   - *Sustained Weight Management*: Beyond initial weight loss, maintaining a hyper ketogenic state can help women keep the weight off, reducing the risk of yo-yo dieting.
2. **Hormonal Balance**
   - *Alleviating PMS Symptoms*: The diet can help stabilize hormonal fluctuations, potentially reducing symptoms like bloating, mood swings, and cravings during the menstrual cycle.
   - *Menopause Management*: Women going through menopause may find relief from symptoms such as hot flashes and night sweats due to the diet's effect on hormone regulation.
3. **Enhanced Mental Clarity and Cognitive Function**
   - *Improved Focus and Concentration*: By providing a steady supply of ketones to the

brain, Hyper Ketosis can enhance cognitive performance, helping women manage demanding work or study schedules.
- *Mood Stabilization*: Some women experience improved mood and reduced anxiety levels, making it easier to handle everyday stressors.

4. **Managing Specific Health Conditions**
   - *Type 2 Diabetes and Insulin Sensitivity*: Reducing carbohydrate intake helps regulate blood sugar levels, which can be particularly beneficial for women with insulin resistance or Type 2 diabetes.
   - *Polycystic Ovary Syndrome (PCOS)*: The diet's impact on reducing insulin levels may aid in managing PCOS symptoms, improving fertility, and regularizing menstrual cycles.

5. **Athletic Performance and Endurance**
   - *Fueling Physical Activity*: Women engaged in endurance sports or high-intensity training might benefit from the sustained energy levels offered by ketones rather than glucose.
   - *Faster Recovery*: The anti-inflammatory effects of ketones can help reduce muscle soreness and speed up recovery times after workouts.

6. **Lifestyle and Well-being**
   - *Increased Energy Levels*: Many women report feeling more energetic and less fatigued

throughout the day, allowing them to juggle work, family, and personal commitments more effectively.
- *Improved Dietary Habits*: Following a Hyper Ketosis diet encourages the consumption of whole foods and healthy fats, promoting a cleaner, more nutritious way of eating.

7. **Long-term Health Benefits**
   - *Cardiovascular Health*: By lowering cholesterol and triglyceride levels, the diet may contribute to improved heart health over time.
   - *Reduced Inflammation*: Chronic inflammation is linked to various health issues; the anti-inflammatory properties of the diet can support overall well-being.

By understanding these use cases, women can tailor the Hyper Ketosis diet to meet their individual health goals and lifestyle needs. As always, consulting with a healthcare provider is advisable to ensure the diet is suitable for one's personal health circumstances.

Principles of the Hyper Ketosis Diet

The hyper ketosis diet is based on the principle of restricting carbohydrates and increasing healthy fat intake to induce the body into a state of ketosis. Some key principles of this diet include:

1. **High Fat, Moderate Protein, Low Carbohydrate Intake**

   The ideal macronutrient ratio for achieving and maintaining a state of ketosis is typically around 75% fat, 20% protein, and a mere 5% carbohydrates. This specific ratio encourages the body to switch from using glucose as its primary energy source to burning fat for fuel, which is essential for those looking to enter and sustain ketosis effectively.

2. **Focus on Whole Foods**

   To achieve optimal nutrition while adhering to this diet, it is crucial to prioritize whole, unprocessed foods. Options such as avocados, which are rich in healthy fats, nuts and seeds that provide essential nutrients, fatty fish like salmon packed with omega-3 fatty acids, and an array of leafy greens loaded with vitamins and minerals should be central to your meal planning. These foods not only support your macronutrient goals but also promote overall health.

3. **Avoid Processed Foods**

   Processed foods are typically high in carbohydrates and often contain unhealthy additives, preservatives, and sugars that can disrupt your ketogenic state. These foods can lead to spikes in blood sugar levels, ultimately hindering your ability to maintain ketosis and possibly leading to unwanted weight gain. Therefore, it's best to avoid packaged snacks, sugary drinks, and any foods with hidden carbs when following a hyper ketosis diet.

4. **Cyclical Ketogenic Diet (CKD)**

   This variation of the hyper ketosis diet introduces periods of higher carbohydrate intake, usually lasting one to two days a week. These "carb-up" days allow the body to replenish its glycogen stores, which can be beneficial for athletes or those undergoing intense physical activity. Additionally, strategically incorporating these carb days can help mitigate potential negative side effects such as fatigue or muscle loss, ensuring that the body continues to operate efficiently while still reaping the benefits of a ketogenic lifestyle.

The principles of the hyper ketosis diet revolve around reducing carbohydrate intake and increasing healthy fat consumption, while also focusing on whole, unprocessed foods for optimal nutrition. It is important to establish an individualized plan with a healthcare professional to determine the best approach for each individual's unique needs and health goals.

5. **Benefits of The Hyper Ketosis Diet**

   While the hyper ketosis diet can benefit individuals of all genders, it may have specific advantages for women's health. Some potential benefits include:

6. **Enhanced Metabolic Health**

   The hyper ketosis diet promotes a significant metabolic shift, encouraging the body to utilize fat as its primary energy source rather than carbohydrates. This shift enhances overall metabolic efficiency, allowing women to manage their energy balance more effectively.

   By restricting carbohydrate intake, the body enters a state of ketosis, where it becomes adept at breaking down fat stores for fuel. This can lead to improved energy levels, better weight management, and a more stable appetite, ultimately supporting a healthier lifestyle. Furthermore, this dietary approach may also contribute to other health benefits, such as improved insulin sensitivity and reduced inflammation.

7. **Increased Fat Burning**

   By entering a deeper state of ketosis, the body significantly enhances fat oxidation processes. This metabolic shift allows women to tap into their stored fat reserves more efficiently, which not only aids in effective weight management but also leads to improved body composition.

As the body becomes more adept at utilizing fat for energy instead of carbohydrates, individuals may experience increased energy levels, reduced cravings, and a greater sense of overall well-being. This holistic approach to fat burning can empower women to achieve their fitness goals and maintain a healthier lifestyle in the long run.

8. Improved Insulin Sensitivity

Reducing carbohydrate intake plays a significant role in stabilizing insulin levels, which can lead to improved insulin sensitivity. By lowering the consumption of refined sugars and high-carb foods, the body becomes more efficient at utilizing insulin, thereby helping to manage blood sugar levels more effectively.

This is particularly important for women, as maintaining balanced insulin levels can reduce the risk of developing insulin resistance, a condition that can disrupt hormonal balance and lead to various health issues. Emphasizing nutrient-dense, low-carbohydrate foods can not only enhance overall metabolic health but also support women's hormonal health by promoting a more stable endocrine environment.

9. **Sustained Energy Levels**

    The consistent production of ketones serves as a reliable and efficient energy source for the body, allowing individuals to avoid the energy crashes often associated with carbohydrate-heavy diets. Unlike glucose, ketones provide a more stable energy supply, which can lead to improved focus and productivity.

    As a result, those following a ketogenic diet often experience sustained energy throughout the day without the peaks and valleys that can make it difficult to stay active and engaged in daily tasks. This stable energy level not only enhances physical performance but also contributes to better mental clarity and overall well-being.

10. **Healthier Skin**

    By reducing oxidative stress and regulating sebum production, the diet can significantly enhance various skin conditions. Oxidative stress can lead to premature aging and skin issues, while balanced sebum levels help prevent clogged pores.

    This combination can contribute to a clearer complexion, reduced acne breakouts, and an overall healthier appearance. Consistently following such a diet may also promote skin elasticity and hydration, providing a youthful glow and minimizing the visibility of blemishes or scars.

These benefits illustrate how the hyper ketosis diet can be a powerful tool for women, addressing their unique health needs and contributing to overall well-being.

Disadvantages of the Hyper Ketosis Diet

While the hyper ketosis diet has its benefits, it is not without its limitations. Some potential disadvantages include:

1. *Initial Fatigue*: Individuals might experience an initial drop in energy levels as their body adapts to burning fat for fuel instead of carbohydrates.
2. *Digestive Changes*: The diet can lead to digestive issues such as constipation due to the sudden increase in fat intake and reduction in fiber-rich foods.
3. *Limited Food Variety*: Adherents might find the restrictive nature of the diet limits their food choices, making it challenging to maintain long-term.
4. *Nutrient Deficiencies*: The absence of certain food groups could result in a lack of essential vitamins and minerals, requiring careful meal planning or supplementation.
5. *Social Challenges*: Dining out and attending social gatherings can become difficult, as menu options may not align with dietary restrictions.

6. ***Keto Flu***: Some may experience flu-like symptoms, known as the "keto flu," during the transition phase, which can include headaches, dizziness, and irritability.

Despite these disadvantages, many find that the health benefits of the Hyper Ketosis Diet, such as improved metabolism and weight loss, outweigh these challenges.

Potential Side Effects of the Hyper Ketosis Diet

In addition to the potential disadvantages, there are also some side effects that individuals may experience while following the hyper ketosis diet. These can include:

1. ***Dehydration***: As carbohydrates are restricted in this diet, it is essential to drink plenty of water and stay hydrated.
2. ***Electrolyte Imbalance***: The reduction in carbohydrate intake can lead to a decrease in electrolytes such as sodium, potassium, and magnesium, which are crucial for proper bodily function.
3. ***Keto Breath***: The production of ketones can result in bad breath or a metallic taste in the mouth.
4. ***Gastrointestinal Issues***: Some individuals may experience digestive issues such as nausea, bloating, or constipation due to the high fat content of the diet.

5. ***Hormonal Changes***: The hyper ketosis diet can affect hormone levels, potentially leading to changes in the menstrual cycle and fertility.

It is essential to be aware of these potential side effects and consult with a healthcare professional before starting the hyper ketosis diet. Additionally, it is recommended to closely monitor any symptoms and adjust the diet accordingly.

5-Step Plan to Get Started with the Hyper Ketosis Diet for Women

Embarking on a hyper ketosis diet can be an exciting journey toward better health and wellness. This diet focuses on significantly reducing carbohydrate intake while increasing fats to help your body enter a state of ketosis, where it burns fat for fuel. Here's a friendly and motivational guide to help you get started on your hyper ketosis journey:

Step 1: Educate Yourself About the Hyper Ketosis Diet

Embarking on the Hyper Ketosis diet requires a solid foundation of knowledge to ensure success and sustainability. By understanding the principles and benefits of ketosis, as well as the dietary components involved, you can make informed decisions that align with your health goals.

Understanding Ketosis

Ketosis is a metabolic state where your body shifts from using carbohydrates as its primary energy source to burning fat. This occurs when carbohydrate intake is significantly reduced, prompting the liver to convert fats into ketones, which serve as an alternative fuel for the body and brain. Grasping the mechanics of ketosis is crucial as it underpins the effectiveness of the Hyper Ketosis diet.

Benefits of Hyper Ketosis

The Hyper Ketosis diet offers numerous benefits, making it an attractive option for many. One of the most notable advantages is increased energy levels. As your body efficiently burns fat, you experience a more consistent and sustained energy supply.

Additionally, many individuals report improved mental clarity, enhanced focus, and better overall cognitive function. These benefits, along with potential weight loss and metabolic improvements, highlight the transformative potential of entering ketosis.

Food Choices in Hyper Ketosis

A successful Hyper Ketosis diet emphasizes the consumption of healthy fats, moderate proteins, and low carbohydrates. Nutrient-dense foods like avocados, nuts, seeds, fatty fish, and olive oil should form the cornerstone of your meals.

Protein sources such as chicken, beef, and eggs are consumed in moderation, while carbohydrate intake is minimized, focusing on non-starchy vegetables.

Understanding these food groups and their roles will help you create balanced meals that support ketosis.

Importance of Knowledge and Commitment

Educating yourself about the Hyper Ketosis diet is not just about understanding the science and food choices; it's about empowering yourself to make informed dietary decisions. With a thorough comprehension of how ketosis works and its benefits, you'll be better positioned to stay committed to the diet. This knowledge acts as a guiding light, helping you navigate challenges and maintain motivation throughout your journey.

By immersing yourself in the intricacies of the Hyper Ketosis diet, you arm yourself with the tools needed to achieve your health and wellness goals.

Step 2: Clean Out Your Pantry

Now that you have a better understanding of the Hyper Ketosis diet, it's time to take action. The next step is to clean out your pantry and remove any temptations that may derail your progress.

Removing High-Carb and Sugary Foods

- *Identify Culprits*: Start by thoroughly identifying and removing foods that are high in carbohydrates and sugars from your pantry and refrigerator. This includes staples such as bread, pasta, and rice, as well as sugary snacks like candies and cookies, and processed foods that often contain hidden sugars. Taking this step is crucial because it sets the foundation for a healthier eating plan and helps you become more mindful of your food choices.

- **Check Labels**: Make it a habit to carefully read food labels for hidden sugars and carbohydrates. Many packaged foods, including condiments, sauces, and even some canned goods, can contain surprising amounts of sugar that you might not expect. Look for terms like high fructose corn syrup, cane sugar, and other sweeteners in the ingredient list, as these can quickly add up and derail your dietary goals.
- **Discard or Donate**: Consider disposing of or donating any non-keto items you discover during your kitchen clean-out. This not only helps you avoid temptation when cravings strike but also frees up space in your kitchen for healthier, keto-friendly options. By creating an environment that supports your dietary choices, you set yourself up for greater success on your health journey.

Stocking Up on Keto-Friendly Staples

1. *Healthy Fats*

Stock your pantry and fridge with a variety of healthy fats, including creamy avocados, crunchy nuts, and nutrient-rich seeds. Incorporate oils like olive and coconut oil, which not only enhance the flavor of your dishes but are also essential for maintaining energy levels and supporting the ketosis process. These fats provide a sustainable source of fuel for your body while promoting overall health.

2. *Proteins*

Make sure to include a diverse range of protein sources in your diet to support muscle growth and repair. Opt for fatty fish like salmon and mackerel, which are packed with omega-3 fatty acids, along with lean meats like chicken and beef. Don't forget about high-quality eggs, which are a versatile and nutrient-dense protein option that can be prepared in numerous ways.

3. *Low-Carb Vegetables*

Maintain a fresh supply of non-starchy vegetables to add variety and essential nutrients to your meals. Leafy greens such as spinach and kale are excellent choices, as they are low in carbs and high in fiber.

Broccoli and zucchini are also great options that provide significant vitamins and minerals while keeping your carb intake in check. These vegetables not only enhance the nutritional profile of your meals but also promote digestive health.

Benefits of Having the Right Foods Available

1. **Ease of Access**

   With a wide variety of keto-friendly foods readily available in stores and online, you'll be much less likely to stray from your dietary goals. Having quick access to the right ingredients not only simplifies meal preparation but also makes snacking more convenient.

   This accessibility allows you to whip up delicious, low-carb meals and snacks without the stress of searching for specific items, ensuring that you stay on track with your keto journey.

2. **Reduced Temptation**

   By consciously eliminating high-carb options from your pantry and fridge, you significantly reduce the chance of making impulsive eating decisions that could derail your progress. This proactive approach helps you avoid the temptation of reaching for quick, unhealthy snacks, allowing you to focus on nourishing your body with keto-approved foods that support your goals.

3. **Encouragement for New Habits**

   A well-stocked pantry filled with keto-friendly ingredients fosters the development of new, healthier eating habits. It encourages you to experiment with different recipes and meal ideas, making the transition to the Hyper Ketosis diet smoother and more sustainable. With a variety of options at your fingertips, you'll find it easier to create nutritious meals that satisfy your cravings while keeping you within your carb limits.

By methodically cleaning out your pantry and restocking with appropriate foods, you create an environment conducive to success on the Hyper Ketosis diet.

Step 3: Plan Your Meals

Effective meal planning is a crucial component of successfully adopting the Hyper Ketosis diet. By creating a structured meal plan, you can ensure nutritional adequacy while minimizing the risk of falling back on high-carb options.

Creating a Balanced Meal Plan

1. *Weekly Planning*

    Dedicate a specific time each week to plan your meals, including breakfast, lunch, dinner, and snacks. Consider creating a meal calendar to visualize your week ahead. This practice helps you stay organized, reduces the stress of last-minute food decisions, and encourages you to choose options that align with your dietary goals. By planning ahead, you can also ensure that you have all the necessary ingredients on hand, making cooking easier and more enjoyable.

2. *Macronutrient Balance*

Ensure that each meal includes a well-thought-out balance of healthy fats, moderate proteins, and low carbohydrates. Healthy fats, such as avocados, nuts, and olive oil, are crucial for supporting overall health and promoting satiety. Moderate protein sources, like lean meats, fish, or plant-based proteins, help with muscle maintenance and repair.

Low carbohydrates, particularly from non-starchy vegetables, are essential for maintaining ketosis, a state that supports fat-burning and provides sustained energy throughout the day. This balanced approach not only fuels your body effectively but also helps maintain mental clarity and focus.

Focus on Easy-to-Prepare Recipes

1. *Simplicity is Key*

When embarking on a new diet, particularly a keto one, it's essential to choose recipes that require minimal ingredients and preparation time. This approach not only streamlines the cooking process but also makes it much easier to adhere to the diet, especially on those particularly busy days when time is of the essence. By focusing on simpler recipes, you can reduce the temptation to reach for unhealthy snacks or convenience foods.

2. Batch Cooking

An excellent strategy for maintaining a keto diet is to prepare larger portions of meals and store them for future use. This not only saves time during the week but also ensures that you always have delicious, keto-friendly options readily available when hunger strikes. Batch cooking can also lead to less food waste, as you can make use of all your ingredients efficiently and enjoy a variety of meals without the daily hassle of cooking.

3. Use of Appliances

Embracing kitchen appliances like slow cookers, air fryers, or pressure cookers can significantly simplify the cooking process while enhancing the flavors of your dishes. These tools allow for hands-off cooking, meaning you can set them up and let them do the work while you focus on other things. Additionally, they can help you prepare meals that retain their taste without the addition of extra carbs, making it easier to stick to your dietary goals while enjoying your food.

4. Ensuring Nutritional Variety

- *Diverse Ingredients*: Incorporate a variety of foods into your meals, including different types of protein such as fish, chicken, legumes, and plant-based options, along with a wide array of vegetables and healthy fats like avocados and nuts. This approach not only prevents meal fatigue by keeping your diet interesting but also ensures that you receive a broad spectrum of essential nutrients that support overall health and wellness.

- *Colorful Plates*: Aim to include a vibrant range of colors in your meals, primarily sourced from fresh vegetables. The more colorful your plate, the higher the likelihood of boosting your intake of vital vitamins and antioxidants. This not only makes your meals visually appealing but also enhances their nutritional value, promoting better health outcomes.

- *Experiment with Flavors*: Don't hesitate to use a variety of herbs and spices to elevate the taste of your dishes without adding extra carbohydrates. Experimenting with different flavor profiles can transform simple meals into culinary delights, making them more enjoyable and satisfying while also adding health benefits through the unique properties of these natural ingredients.

5. ***Importance of Meal Planning***
    - *Avoiding Temptations*: With a well-thought-out plan in place, you're significantly less likely to resort to carb-heavy, off-diet foods that can derail your progress. By having meals prepped and ready to go, you not only reduce the likelihood of impulsively ordering takeout but also eliminate the urge to grab unhealthy snacks that may be lurking in your pantry. This proactive approach makes it easier to stick to your dietary goals and ultimately promotes a healthier lifestyle.

    - *Nutritional Assurance*: Proper meal planning is crucial as it ensures that you consistently meet your nutritional needs without the guesswork. By carefully selecting ingredients and portion sizes, you can support your overall health while effectively functioning on the Hyper Ketosis diet. This structured approach allows you to incorporate a variety of nutrients, which is essential for maintaining energy levels and overall well-being during ketosis.

    - *Consistency and Commitment*: Adopting a structured approach to your meals fosters consistency in your eating habits, which is vital for achieving long-term success. When you commit to a meal plan, you're better equipped to stay on track with your dietary goals. This discipline not only maximizes the benefits offered by the Hyper Ketosis diet but also builds a strong foundation for sustainable eating habits that can lead to lasting health improvements.

By dedicating time to plan your meals, you set yourself up for a successful transition into and maintenance of the Hyper Ketosis lifestyle, ensuring that both your nutritional needs and taste preferences are met.

Step 4: Track Your Progress

Tracking your progress on the Hyper Ketosis diet is a powerful tool for maintaining motivation and ensuring you stay on the right path. By systematically documenting your journey, you gain insights into your habits and make informed adjustments as needed.

Using Journals or Apps

- *Choosing a Method*: When starting your journaling journey, take the time to decide whether you prefer a physical journal or a digital app. Both options come with distinct advantages—physical journals offer a personal touch, allowing you to express your creativity through handwritten entries and sketches, while digital apps provide convenience, easy accessibility, and automated features that can simplify the process.

- *Features to Look For*: If you opt for a digital app, make sure to find one that allows for comprehensive tracking. Look for features that enable you to log meals, track your exercise routines, monitor your mood, and even set goals. This holistic approach will not only give you a clearer picture of your progress but also help you identify patterns and make informed decisions about your lifestyle choices.

- *Consistency is Key*: No matter which method you ultimately choose for your journaling, maintaining consistency in logging your daily experiences is crucial. Regular entries will help you gather reliable data over time, enabling you to reflect on your journey and make adjustments as needed for continuous improvement. Remember, the more consistent you are, the more meaningful insights you will gain from your journaling practice.

Documenting Meals and Feelings

- *Meal Logging*: Keeping detailed records of what you eat, including portion sizes and ingredients, is crucial for understanding your dietary habits. This practice not only helps you track calorie intake but also allows you to identify patterns that could significantly impact your progress toward your health goals. By reviewing your logs, you might discover certain foods or meal times that lead to weight gain or other health issues.

- ***Emotional Tracking***: It's important to note how you feel physically and mentally each day. This daily reflection can uncover correlations between your dietary choices and your mood or energy levels. For instance, you may find that certain foods lift your spirits while others leave you feeling sluggish or irritable. Understanding these connections can empower you to make healthier choices that enhance your overall well-being.

- ***Identify Triggers***: Documenting your feelings can be a powerful tool in identifying emotional or situational triggers that lead to cravings or dietary lapses. By recognizing times when you're more likely to indulge in unhealthy foods—whether due to stress, boredom, or social situations—you can develop strategies to cope with these triggers more effectively. This awareness can help you make better choices at the moment, ultimately supporting your long-term health goals.

Tracking Physical Changes

- *Weight and Measurements*: Regularly record your weight and body measurements. This provides tangible evidence of your progress and highlights areas of success.

- *Visual Progress*: Consider taking progress photos at regular intervals to visually capture changes over time. This can be incredibly motivating when the scale doesn't tell the full story.

- *Performance Metrics*: Track improvements in physical activities, such as increased stamina or strength, as these are also significant indicators of progress.

Benefits of Monitoring Progress

- *Motivational Boost*: Seeing documented progress can significantly boost your motivation, reinforcing your commitment to the diet.
- *Adjustments and Tweaks*: Regular tracking allows you to spot trends and make necessary adjustments to your diet or lifestyle to continue progressing.
- *Accountability*: Keeping a consistent record holds you accountable to your goals, providing a sense of responsibility toward maintaining your dietary commitments.

Importance of Regular Review

- *Weekly Reviews*: Set aside time weekly to review your entries. Reflect on what's working and what might need change.
- *Goal Setting*: Use your tracking data to set new goals or refine existing ones, ensuring they are realistic and aligned with your desired outcomes.
- *Celebrate Milestones*: Acknowledge and celebrate achievements, big or small, to maintain enthusiasm and dedication.

By diligently tracking your progress on the Hyper Ketosis diet, you empower yourself with the knowledge needed to stay focused and achieve lasting results.

Step 5: Stay Motivated and Adjust as Needed

Maintaining motivation while following the Hyper Ketosis diet is crucial for long-term success. Embrace the journey with a positive mindset and be prepared to make adjustments as needed to sustain progress.

Celebrating Small Victories

- *Acknowledge Achievements*: Regularly celebrate your progress, whether it's reaching a weight milestone or sticking to your meal plan for a week. These small victories keep you motivated and reinforce positive behaviors.

- ***Reward System***: Set up a reward system to achieve your goals. Rewards could range from a new workout outfit to a relaxing day out. Ensure they align with your health goals and encourage continued progress.

Setting Realistic Goals

- ***SMART Goals***: Set Specific, Measurable, Achievable, Relevant, and Time-bound goals to provide clear direction. This approach makes it easier to track progress and maintain focus.
- ***Short and Long-Term Goals***: Balance short-term objectives with long-term aspirations to keep motivation high and provide a roadmap for sustained success.

Finding Support

- ***Join Communities***: Engage with online forums or local groups dedicated to the Hyper Ketosis diet. Sharing experiences and challenges with like-minded individuals provides support and inspiration.
- ***Accountability Partners***: Consider partnering with a friend or family member who shares similar health goals. Mutual encouragement and accountability can significantly boost motivation.

Being Open to Adjustments

- *Listen to Your Body*: Understand that each body responds differently to dietary changes. Stay attuned to how your body feels and be ready to adjust your diet if necessary.
- *Consult Professionals*: If you're unsure about adjustments, consider seeking advice from nutritionists or dietitians who specialize in ketosis. Professional guidance can ensure you're making informed changes.

Emphasizing Patience and a Positive Mindset

- *Stay Patient*: Remember that significant changes take time. Be patient with your progress and avoid comparing yourself to others.
- *Positive Affirmations*: Use positive affirmations to maintain a healthy mindset. Remind yourself of your strengths and the reasons you embarked on this journey.
- *Focus on the Journey*: Enjoy the process of transforming your health, recognizing that each step brings you closer to a healthier, more energized you.

By embracing these strategies, you can maintain motivation and make necessary adjustments to the Hyper Ketosis diet, ensuring a successful and sustainable journey towards better health.

Tips for Success

- ***Stay Hydrated***: Drinking plenty of water is vital for overall health, especially during ketosis, as it can have a diuretic effect that leads to increased fluid loss. Aim for at least 8-10 glasses of water a day, and consider including electrolyte-rich beverages to help maintain balance.
- ***Watch Out for the Keto Flu***: When transitioning to a ketogenic diet, you may encounter symptoms commonly referred to as the "keto flu," which can include fatigue, headaches, irritability, and nausea. To combat these symptoms, ensure you're consuming enough electrolytes, such as sodium, potassium, and magnesium, which can help ease the transition.
- ***Be Patient***: It's important to remember that achieving results on a ketogenic diet can take time, as your body needs to adjust to burning fat for fuel instead of carbohydrates. Be patient with this adjustment process, and don't get discouraged if you don't see immediate changes; consistency is key.
- ***Consult Professionals***: If you're unsure about how to structure your ketogenic diet, consider seeking advice from a nutritionist or dietitian who can help tailor the plan to your specific needs and dietary preferences. They can provide personalized guidance and ensure you're meeting your nutritional requirements while following the diet.

By following these steps, you'll be well on your way to successfully embracing the hyper ketosis lifestyle. Stay positive, stay informed, and enjoy the journey to a healthier you!

Foods to Eat

Including a balance of the following nutrient-dense foods in your diet can support the Hyper Ketosis Diet and optimize physical performance:

- *Avocados*: Rich in healthy fats and low in carbs, avocados are ideal for maintaining ketosis while providing essential nutrients like potassium.
- *Nuts and Seeds*: Almonds, walnuts, and chia seeds are excellent sources of healthy fats, fiber, and protein, making them perfect snacks or additions to meals.
- *Fatty Fish*: Salmon, mackerel, and sardines are high in omega-3 fatty acids, which support heart health and aid in fat metabolism.
- *Oils*: Olive oil, coconut oil, and avocado oil are great for cooking or dressing salads, offering high-fat content to help sustain ketosis.
- *Cheese*: Most types of cheese are low in carbs and high in fat, making them a tasty and satisfying choice for the diet.

- ***Leafy Greens***: Spinach, kale, and arugula are low in carbs but rich in vitamins and minerals, essential for maintaining overall health.

By incorporating these foods into your meals, you can create a well-rounded and sustainable diet that supports the Hyper Ketosis Diet and promotes optimal health.

Foods to Avoid

To maintain ketosis and achieve success with the Hyper Ketosis Diet, it's important to limit or avoid foods containing high levels of carbohydrates. These include:

- ***Bread and Pasta***: High-carb foods like bread and pasta can quickly knock you out of ketosis and should be replaced with low-carb alternatives.
- ***Sugary Snacks***: Items like candy, cookies, and cakes are loaded with sugar, which spikes insulin levels and disrupts ketosis.
- ***Starchy Vegetables***: Potatoes, corn, and peas are high in carbs and should be avoided or consumed in very limited quantities.
- ***Sweetened Beverages***: Drinks like soda and juice are high in sugar and can easily exceed your daily carb limit, hindering ketosis.
- ***Grains***: Rice, oats, and quinoa are high in carbohydrates and should be replaced with low-carb options to maintain ketosis.

- ***Legumes***: Beans and lentils are relatively high in carbs and can interfere with maintaining a ketogenic state.

By limiting or avoiding these foods, you can better support your body's transition into ketosis and reap the benefits of the Hyper Ketosis Diet.

7-Day Sample Meal Plan

Now that you have a better understanding of what foods to include and exclude on the Hyper Ketosis Diet, here is a sample 7-day meal plan to help get you started:

Day 1

Breakfast: Spinach and feta omelet with avocado slices

Lunch: Grilled chicken salad with mixed greens, bell peppers, and olive oil dressing

Dinner: Baked salmon with broccoli and cauliflower rice

Day 2

Breakfast: Bacon and eggs with sliced tomatoes

Lunch: Tuna salad wrap made with low-carb tortilla and lettuce

Dinner: Beef stir-fry with vegetables over zucchini noodles

Day 3

Breakfast: Greek yogurt with mixed berries and almonds

Lunch: Turkey and cheese roll-ups with cucumber slices

Dinner: Baked chicken thighs with roasted Brussels sprouts and mushrooms

Day 4

Breakfast: Keto-friendly granola with almond milk

Lunch: Zucchini noodles with shrimp scampi

Dinner: Grilled pork chops with asparagus and garlic butter sauce

Day 5

Breakfast: Avocado toast made with low-carb bread and topped with smoked salmon

Lunch: Caesar salad with grilled chicken breast

Dinner: Spaghetti squash bolognese topped with Parmesan cheese

Day 6

Breakfast: Ham and cheese omelet with sautéed mushrooms

Lunch: Tofu and vegetable stir-fry with soy sauce

Dinner: Baked cod with roasted cauliflower and zucchini

Day 7

Breakfast: Keto-friendly pancakes topped with sugar-free syrup and berries

Lunch: Chicken Caesar wrap made with low-carb tortilla and romaine lettuce

Dinner: Beef fajita bowl with avocado, sour cream, and salsa

Sample Recipes

Now that you have a general idea of what meals to include in your ketogenic meal plan, here are some sample recipes to try out:

Keto-Friendly Pancakes

Ingredients:

- 1 cup almond flour
- 2 large eggs
- 1/4 cup coconut milk (unsweetened)
- 1 tablespoon coconut oil (melted)
- 1 teaspoon vanilla extract
- 1/2 teaspoon baking powder
- A pinch of salt
- Butter or coconut oil for cooking

Toppings:

- Sugar-free syrup
- Fresh berries (such as raspberries and blueberries)

Instructions:

1. Prepare the Batter:
2. In a mixing bowl, combine almond flour, baking powder, and a pinch of salt. Stir to mix the dry ingredients.
3. In another bowl, whisk together the eggs, coconut milk, melted coconut oil, and vanilla extract until well combined.
4. Gradually add the wet ingredients to the dry ingredients, mixing until you have a smooth batter. Let the batter sit for a few minutes to thicken.

Cook the Pancakes:

5. Heat a non-stick skillet over medium heat and add a small amount of butter or coconut oil to coat the pan.
6. Pour about 1/4 cup of batter onto the skillet for each pancake. Cook for 2-3 minutes or until bubbles form on the surface and the edges look set.
7. Carefully flip the pancake and cook for an additional 2-3 minutes until golden brown.
8. Repeat with the remaining batter, adding more butter or oil to the skillet as needed.

Serve:

9. Stack the pancakes on a plate and drizzle with sugar-free syrup.
10. Top with a handful of fresh raspberries and blueberries for a burst of flavor and color.
11. Serving Size: This recipe makes about four pancakes, the perfect portion size for a satisfying breakfast or brunch for women following the Hyper Ketosis Diet.

Chicken Caesar Wrap

Ingredients:

- 2 low-carb tortillas
- 1 cup grilled chicken breast, sliced
- 2 tablespoons Caesar dressing (sugar-free)
- 2 tablespoons grated Parmesan cheese
- 1 cup romaine lettuce, chopped
- 1/4 avocado, sliced (optional)
- Salt and pepper to taste
- Olive oil for grilling

Instructions:

Grill the Chicken:

1. Season the chicken breast with salt and pepper. Heat a grill pan over medium-high heat and add a drizzle of olive oil.
2. Grill the chicken for about 5-6 minutes on each side, or until fully cooked and golden brown.
3. Remove from heat and let it rest for a few minutes before slicing.

Prepare the Wrap:

4. Lay out the low-carb tortillas on a clean surface.
5. Spread 1 tablespoon of Caesar dressing on each tortilla for flavor.

Assemble the Ingredients:

6. Evenly distribute the chopped romaine lettuce over each tortilla.
7. Add the grilled chicken slices on top of the lettuce.
8. Sprinkle 1 tablespoon of Parmesan cheese over each wrap.
9. Add avocado slices for extra creaminess and healthy fats, if desired.

Wrap It Up:

10. Carefully roll the tortilla, tucking in the sides as you go to create a snug wrap.
11. Slice each wrap in half for easy serving.

Serving Size: This recipe makes two wraps, perfect for a satisfying lunch or dinner for those following the Hyper Ketosis Diet.

Beef Fajita Bowl

Ingredients:

- 1 pound beef strips (such as flank steak or sirloin)
- 1 tablespoon olive oil
- 1 red bell pepper, sliced
- 1 green bell pepper, sliced
- 1 medium onion, sliced
- 1 teaspoon garlic powder
- 1 teaspoon cumin
- 1 teaspoon chili powder
- Salt and pepper to taste
- 1 avocado, sliced
- 1/2 cup sour cream
- 1/2 cup salsa (sugar-free)
- Fresh cilantro for garnish (optional)

Instructions:

Prepare the Beef:

1. In a large skillet over medium-high heat, add olive oil.
2. Season the beef strips with garlic powder, cumin, chili powder, salt, and pepper.
3. Add the beef strips to the skillet and cook for 5-7 minutes, or until they are browned and cooked to your desired level of doneness. Remove from the skillet and set aside.

Cook the Vegetables:

4. In the same skillet, add a little more olive oil if needed.
5. Add the sliced bell peppers and onion. Cook for about 5 minutes, stirring occasionally, until the vegetables are tender and slightly charred.

Assemble the Fajita Bowl:

6. Divide the cooked beef and vegetables between serving bowls.
7. Top each bowl with avocado slices, a dollop of sour cream, and salsa.
8. Garnish with fresh cilantro if desired.

Serving Size: This recipe serves approximately 4, making it a perfect ketogenic meal option for lunch or dinner.

Ham and Cheese Omelet with Sautéed Mushrooms

Ingredients:

- 3 large eggs
- 1/4 cup diced ham
- 1/4 cup shredded cheddar cheese
- 1/2 cup mushrooms, sliced
- 1 tablespoon butter
- Salt and pepper to taste
- Fresh parsley for garnish (optional)

Instructions:

Prepare the Mushrooms:

1. In a small skillet, melt half of the butter over medium heat.
2. Add the sliced mushrooms and sauté for about 5 minutes, or until they are tender and golden brown. Set aside.

Make the Omelet:

3. In a bowl, whisk the eggs with a pinch of salt and pepper until well combined.
4. In a non-stick skillet, melt the remaining butter over medium-low heat.
5. Pour in the beaten eggs, tilting the skillet to evenly distribute the mixture.

6. Cook gently, using a spatula to lift the edges, and allow uncooked eggs to flow underneath.

Add the Filling:

7. Once the omelet is mostly set but still slightly runny on top, sprinkle the diced ham and shredded cheese over one-half.
8. Add the sautéed mushrooms on top of the ham and cheese.

Fold and Serve:

9. Carefully fold the omelet in half to cover the filling. Cook for another minute or until the cheese is melted and the omelet is fully set.
10. Slide the omelet onto a plate and garnish with fresh parsley if desired.

Serving Size: This recipe makes one generous omelet, perfect for a hearty breakfast or brunch on the Hyper Ketosis Diet.

Tofu and Vegetable Stir-Fry

Ingredients:

- 1 block (14 oz) firm tofu, drained and cubed
- 2 tablespoons soy sauce (low sodium)
- 1 tablespoon sesame oil
- 1 tablespoon olive oil
- 1 cup broccoli florets
- 1 red bell pepper, sliced
- 1 cup zucchini, sliced
- 1/2 cup snap peas
- 2 cloves garlic, minced
- 1 teaspoon ginger, grated
- Sesame seeds for garnish (optional)
- Salt and pepper to taste

Instructions:

Prepare the Tofu:

1. Press the tofu to remove excess moisture by wrapping it in a clean kitchen towel and placing a heavy object on top for about 15 minutes.
2. Cut the tofu into bite-sized cubes.

Marinate the Tofu:

3. In a bowl, mix the tofu cubes with 1 tablespoon of soy sauce and let it marinate for 10 minutes.

Cook the Tofu:

4. In a large skillet or wok, heat the olive oil over medium-high heat.
5. Add the marinated tofu cubes and cook until they are golden brown on all sides, about 5-7 minutes. Remove the tofu from the skillet and set aside.

Stir-Fry the Vegetables:

6. In the same skillet, add sesame oil. Once hot, add garlic and ginger, stirring for about 30 seconds until fragrant.
7. Add broccoli, bell pepper, zucchini, and snap peas. Stir-fry for 4-5 minutes, or until the vegetables are tender-crisp.

Combine and Season:

8. Return the tofu to the skillet with the vegetables.
9. Add the remaining tablespoon of soy sauce and stir everything together, cooking for another 2 minutes to heat through.
10. Season with salt and pepper to taste.

Serve:

11. Divide the stir-fry into servings and garnish with sesame seeds if desired.

Serving Size: This recipe makes about 4 servings, perfect for a healthy and satisfying meal on the Hyper Ketosis Diet.

Baked Cod

Ingredients:

- 4 fresh cod filets (about 6 oz each)
- 1 medium cauliflower, cut into florets
- 2 medium zucchinis, sliced into half-moons
- 3 tablespoons olive oil
- 1 teaspoon garlic powder
- 1 teaspoon onion powder
- 1 teaspoon dried thyme
- Salt and pepper to taste
- Lemon wedges for serving
- Fresh parsley for garnish (optional)

Instructions:

Preheat the Oven:

1. Preheat your oven to 400°F (200°C).

Prepare the Vegetables:

2. In a large bowl, toss the cauliflower florets and zucchini slices with 2 tablespoons of olive oil, garlic powder, onion powder, salt, and pepper.
3. Spread the vegetables evenly on a baking sheet lined with parchment paper.

Roast the Vegetables:

4. Place the baking sheet in the oven and roast the vegetables for about 20-25 minutes, or until they are tender and slightly golden, stirring halfway through.

Prepare the Cod:

5. While the vegetables are roasting, pat the cod filets dry with paper towels and season both sides with salt, pepper, and dried thyme.
6. Drizzle the remaining tablespoon of olive oil over the cod filets.

Bake the Cod:

7. Once the vegetables have cooked for 25 minutes, remove the baking sheet from the oven and make space for the cod filets.
8. Place the cod filets on the baking sheet alongside the vegetables.
9. Return the baking sheet to the oven and bake for an additional 10-15 minutes, or until the cod is opaque and flakes easily with a fork.

Serve:

10. Transfer the baked cod and roasted vegetables to plates.
11. Garnish with fresh parsley and serve with lemon wedges on the side.

Serving Size: This recipe serves 4, making it an ideal ketogenic meal option for lunch or dinner.

Avocado Toast with Smoked Salmon on Low-Carb Bread

Ingredients:

- 2 slices of low-carb bread
- 1 ripe avocado
- 1 tablespoon lemon juice
- Salt and pepper to taste
- 4 ounces smoked salmon
- 1 tablespoon capers (optional)
- Fresh dill for garnish (optional)
- Red pepper flakes for a kick (optional)

Instructions:

Prepare the Avocado Spread:

1. Cut the avocado in half, remove the pit, and scoop the flesh into a bowl.
2. Add the lemon juice, salt, and pepper. Mash with a fork until you reach your desired consistency.

Toast the Bread:

3. Toast the slices of low-carb bread to your liking.
4. Assemble the Avocado Toast:
5. Spread the mashed avocado evenly over each slice of toasted bread.

Add the Smoked Salmon:

6. Lay the smoked salmon slices on top of the avocado spread.

Finish with Toppings:

7. Sprinkle capers over the top if using.
8. Garnish with fresh dill and a pinch of red pepper flakes for extra flavor, if desired.

Serving Size: This recipe serves 2, making it a perfect breakfast or light meal option for those on the Hyper Ketosis Diet.

Caesar Salad with Grilled Chicken Breast

Ingredients:

- 2 large chicken breasts
- 1 tablespoon olive oil
- Salt and pepper to taste
- 1 teaspoon garlic powder
- 1 large head of romaine lettuce, chopped
- 1/2 cup Caesar dressing (low-carb)
- 1/4 cup grated Parmesan cheese
- 1/4 cup almond slivers or keto-friendly croutons
- Lemon wedges for serving
- Fresh parsley for garnish (optional)

Instructions:

Prepare the Chicken:

1. Preheat your grill to medium-high heat.
2. Brush the chicken breasts with olive oil and season with salt, pepper, and garlic powder.

Grill the Chicken:

3. Place the chicken breasts on the grill. Cook for about 6-7 minutes on each side, or until the internal temperature reaches 165°F (75°C) and the chicken is no longer pink inside.
4. Once cooked, remove the chicken from the grill and let it rest for a few minutes before slicing.

Prepare the Salad:

5. While the chicken is resting, place the chopped romaine lettuce in a large salad bowl.
6. Drizzle the Caesar dressing over the lettuce and toss until evenly coated.

Assemble the Salad:

7. Slice the grilled chicken breasts and arrange them over the dressed lettuce.
8. Sprinkle with grated Parmesan cheese and almond slivers or keto-friendly croutons.

Garnish and Serve:

9. Add lemon wedges on the side for a fresh squeeze of citrus flavor.
10. Garnish with fresh parsley if desired.

Serving Size: This recipe makes approximately 2 servings, making it a hearty and delicious option for lunch or dinner on the Hyper Ketosis Diet.

Spaghetti Squash Bolognese

Ingredients:

- 1 medium spaghetti squash
- 1 pound ground beef
- 2 tablespoons olive oil
- 1 small onion, finely chopped
- 2 cloves garlic, minced
- 1 can (14 oz) low-carb tomato sauce
- 1 teaspoon dried oregano
- 1 teaspoon dried basil
- Salt and pepper to taste
- 1/2 cup grated Parmesan cheese
- Fresh parsley for garnish (optional)

Instructions:

Prepare the Spaghetti Squash:

1. Preheat your oven to 400°F (200°C).
2. Cut the spaghetti squash in half lengthwise and scoop out the seeds.
3. Drizzle the inside with 1 tablespoon of olive oil and season with salt and pepper.
4. Place the squash halves cut-side down on a baking sheet lined with parchment paper.
5. Bake for 30-40 minutes, or until the squash is tender and easily shredded with a fork.

Cook the Bolognese Sauce:

6. While the squash is baking, heat the remaining tablespoon of olive oil in a large skillet over medium heat.
7. Add the chopped onion and garlic, sautéing until the onion is translucent.
8. Add the ground beef to the skillet, cooking until browned and cooked through. Drain excess fat if necessary.
9. Stir in the tomato sauce, oregano, basil, salt, and pepper. Simmer for 15-20 minutes, allowing the flavors to meld.

Assemble the Dish:

10. Once the spaghetti squash is cooked, use a fork to scrape out the strands into a large serving bowl.
11. Pour the Bolognese sauce over the spaghetti squash strands and toss gently to combine.

Serve:

12. Divide the spaghetti squash Bolognese into servings and top each with a generous sprinkle of Parmesan cheese.
13. Garnish with fresh parsley if desired.

Serving Size: This recipe makes about 4 servings, making it a satisfying and delicious meal option for those on the Hyper Ketosis Diet.

Keto-Friendly Granola with Almond Milk

Ingredients:

- 1 cup almonds, roughly chopped
- 1 cup pecans, roughly chopped
- 1/2 cup pumpkin seeds
- 1/2 cup sunflower seeds
- 1/2 cup unsweetened coconut flakes
- 2 tablespoons chia seeds
- 2 tablespoons flaxseed meal
- 1/4 cup coconut oil, melted
- 1/4 cup keto-friendly sweetener (such as erythritol or monk fruit)
- 1 teaspoon vanilla extract
- 1 teaspoon cinnamon
- 1/4 teaspoon salt

Instructions:

Preheat the Oven:

1. Preheat your oven to 325°F (165°C).
2. Line a baking sheet with parchment paper.

Combine Dry Ingredients:

3. In a large mixing bowl, combine the almonds, pecans, pumpkin seeds, sunflower seeds, coconut flakes, chia seeds, and flaxseed meal. Stir well to ensure even distribution.

Prepare the Wet Mixture:

4. In a small saucepan over low heat, melt the coconut oil. Remove from heat and stir in the keto-friendly sweetener, vanilla extract, cinnamon, and salt until well combined.

Mix Together:

5. Pour the wet mixture over the dry ingredients. Stir thoroughly to coat all the ingredients evenly.

Bake the Granola:

6. Spread the granola mixture evenly on the prepared baking sheet.
7. Bake for 20-25 minutes, stirring halfway through, until golden brown and fragrant.
8. Keep an eye on it to prevent burning.

Cool and Store:

9. Remove from the oven and allow the granola to cool completely on the baking sheet.
10. Once cooled, transfer to an airtight container for storage.

Serving Size: This recipe makes approximately 8 servings. Serve with unsweetened almond milk for a delicious keto-friendly breakfast or snack.

Zucchini Noodles with Shrimp Scampi

Ingredients:

- 4 medium zucchinis, spiralized into noodles
- 1 pound large shrimp, peeled and deveined
- 3 tablespoons butter
- 3 cloves garlic, minced
- 1/4 cup chicken broth or white wine
- 2 tablespoons lemon juice
- Salt and pepper to taste
- 1/4 teaspoon red pepper flakes (optional)
- 2 tablespoons chopped fresh parsley
- Lemon wedges for serving

Instructions:

Prepare the Zucchini Noodles:

1. Use a spiralizer to create noodles from the zucchini. Set aside.

Cook the Shrimp:

2. In a large skillet, melt 2 tablespoons of butter over medium heat.
3. Add the garlic and sauté until fragrant, about 1 minute.
4. Add the shrimp to the skillet, and season with salt, pepper, and red pepper flakes if using. Cook for about 2-3 minutes on each side, or until the shrimp are pink and opaque.

5. Remove the shrimp from the skillet and set aside.

Make the Scampi Sauce:

6. In the same skillet, add the remaining tablespoon of butter.
7. Pour in the chicken broth or white wine, and lemon juice, stirring to combine. Bring the mixture to a simmer.

Cook the Zucchini Noodles:

8. Add the zucchini noodles to the skillet, tossing them in the sauce for about 2-3 minutes, or until they're slightly softened but still firm (al dente).

Combine and Serve:

9. Return the cooked shrimp to the skillet. Toss everything together to coat the shrimp and noodles in the sauce.
10. Sprinkle with chopped parsley before serving.

Serving Size: This recipe makes about 4 servings, making it a light and flavorful meal option for those on the Hyper Ketosis Diet.

Grilled Pork Chops with Asparagus and Garlic Butter Sauce

Ingredients:

- 4 bone-in pork chops (about 1-inch thick)
- 1 pound fresh asparagus, trimmed
- 4 tablespoons butter
- 3 cloves garlic, minced
- 1 tablespoon olive oil
- Salt and pepper to taste
- 1 teaspoon dried thyme
- Lemon wedges for serving

Instructions:

Prepare the Grill:

1. Preheat your grill to medium-high heat.

Season the Pork Chops:

2. Pat the pork chops dry with paper towels.
3. Rub both sides with olive oil and season generously with salt, pepper, and dried thyme.

Grill the Pork Chops:

4. Place the pork chops on the grill and cook for about 4-5 minutes on each side, or until they reach an internal temperature of 145°F (63°C).

5. Remove from the grill and let them rest for a few minutes.

Prepare the Asparagus:

6. While the pork chops are grilling, toss the asparagus with a bit of olive oil, salt, and pepper.
7. Place the asparagus on the grill and cook for about 3-4 minutes, turning occasionally, until tender and slightly charred.

Make the Garlic Butter Sauce:

8. In a small saucepan, melt the butter over medium heat.
9. Add the minced garlic and cook until fragrant, about 1-2 minutes. Be careful not to burn the garlic.
10. Remove from heat and set aside.

Serve:

11. Drizzle the garlic butter sauce over the grilled pork chops and asparagus.
12. Serve with lemon wedges for an extra burst of flavor.

Serving Size: This recipe makes about 4 servings, making it a hearty and delicious option for those on the Hyper Ketosis Diet.

Turkey and Cheese Roll-Ups with Cucumber Slices

Ingredients:

- 8 slices of turkey breast
- 8 slices of cheddar or Swiss cheese
- 1 large cucumber
- 2 tablespoons cream cheese (optional)
- Salt and pepper to taste
- Fresh dill or parsley for garnish (optional)

Instructions:

Prepare the Cucumber:

1. Wash the cucumber thoroughly and pat it dry.
2. Using a sharp knife or a mandoline, slice the cucumber into thin rounds. Sprinkle with a pinch of salt and pepper to taste.

Assemble the Roll-Ups:

3. Lay a slice of turkey breast flat on a clean surface.
4. Place a slice of cheese on top of the turkey. If using cream cheese, spread a thin layer over the cheese.
5. Starting from one end, gently roll the turkey and cheese into a tight cylinder.

Secure and Serve:

6. Optionally, secure each roll-up with a toothpick.

7. Arrange the turkey and cheese roll-ups on a serving platter alongside the cucumber slices.
8. Garnish with fresh dill or parsley for added flair if desired.

Serving Size: This recipe makes approximately 4 servings, providing a quick and tasty meal or snack option for those following the Hyper Ketosis Diet.

Baked Chicken Thighs

Ingredients:

- 6 bone-in, skin-on chicken thighs
- 1 pound Brussels sprouts, halved
- 8 ounces mushrooms, quartered
- 3 tablespoons olive oil
- 1 tablespoon balsamic vinegar
- 3 cloves garlic, minced
- 1 teaspoon dried rosemary
- 1 teaspoon dried thyme
- Salt and pepper to taste
- Fresh parsley for garnish (optional)

Instructions:

Preheat the Oven:

1. Preheat your oven to 400°F (200°C).

Prepare the Chicken Thighs:

2. Pat the chicken thighs dry with paper towels.
3. Season generously with salt, pepper, rosemary, and thyme on both sides.

Prepare the Vegetables:

4. In a large bowl, combine the Brussels sprouts and mushrooms.

5. Add the olive oil, balsamic vinegar, minced garlic, salt, and pepper. Toss to coat the vegetables evenly.

Assemble in Baking Dish:

6. Arrange the seasoned chicken thighs in a single layer on a large baking sheet or dish.
7. Surround the chicken with the Brussels sprouts and mushrooms.

Bake:

8. Place the baking dish in the oven and bake for 35-45 minutes, or until the chicken reaches an internal temperature of 165°F (74°C) and is golden brown.
9. Stir the vegetables halfway through cooking to ensure even roasting.

Serve:

10. Transfer the chicken and vegetables to a serving platter.
11. Garnish with fresh parsley if desired.

Serving Size: This recipe makes about 4 servings, providing a hearty and flavorful meal for those on the Hyper Ketosis Diet.

Tuna Salad Wrap

Ingredients:

- 2 cans (5 oz each) of tuna in water, drained
- 1/4 cup mayonnaise
- 1 tablespoon Dijon mustard
- 1 stalk celery, finely chopped
- 1/4 cup red onion, finely chopped
- 1 tablespoon fresh lemon juice
- Salt and pepper to taste
- 4 low-carb tortillas
- 4 large lettuce leaves (romaine or iceberg)
- 1/4 cup sliced olives (optional)
- Fresh dill or parsley for garnish (optional)

Instructions:

Prepare the Tuna Salad:

1. Mix the drained tuna, mayonnaise, Dijon mustard, celery, red onion, and lemon juice together in a medium-sized bowl.
2. Mix well until all ingredients are thoroughly combined.
3. Season with salt and pepper to taste.

Assemble the Wraps:

4. Lay a low-carb tortilla flat on a clean surface.
5. Place a lettuce leaf in the center of the tortilla.

6. Spoon a portion of the tuna salad onto the lettuce leaf.
7. Add a few sliced olives for additional flavor, if desired.

Roll the Wraps:

8. Fold the sides of the tortilla over the filling.
9. Starting from the bottom, roll the tortilla tightly into a wrap.
10. Repeat the process with the remaining tortillas and tuna salad.

Serve:

11. Cut each wrap in half for easier handling.
12. Arrange on a serving platter and garnish with fresh dill or parsley, if desired.

Serving Size: This recipe makes approximately 4 wraps, making it a convenient and tasty meal for those following the Hyper Ketosis Diet.

Beef Stir-Fry with Vegetables over Zucchini Noodles

Ingredients:

- 1 pound beef strips (sirloin or flank steak)
- 4 medium zucchinis, spiralized into noodles
- 1 red bell pepper, sliced
- 1 cup broccoli florets
- 1 cup sliced mushrooms
- 1/2 cup snow peas
- 3 tablespoons coconut oil or avocado oil
- 3 cloves garlic, minced
- 1 tablespoon ginger, grated
- 2 tablespoons soy sauce or tamari (for a gluten-free option)
- 1 tablespoon rice vinegar
- Salt and pepper to taste
- Sesame seeds and sliced green onions for garnish (optional)

Instructions:

Prepare the Zucchini Noodles:

1. Spiralize the zucchini into noodles and set aside.
2. In a large pan over medium heat, add 1 tablespoon of oil.

3. Add the zucchini noodles and sauté for 2-3 minutes until slightly softened. Season with a pinch of salt. Remove from heat and set aside.

Cook the Beef:

4. In the same pan, add another tablespoon of oil.
5. Add the beef strips, season with salt and pepper, and cook over high heat until browned on all sides, about 4-5 minutes. Remove the beef from the pan and set aside.

Stir-Fry the Vegetables:

1. Add the remaining tablespoon of oil to the pan.
2. Add the garlic and ginger, and sauté for about 30 seconds until fragrant.
3. Add the bell pepper, broccoli, mushrooms, and snow peas. Stir-fry for 5-6 minutes until the vegetables are tender-crisp.

Combine and Season:

4. Return the beef to the pan with the vegetables.
5. Add the soy sauce and rice vinegar. Stir well to combine all ingredients and heat through.

Serve:

6. Divide the zucchini noodles among four plates.
7. Top each plate with the beef and vegetable stir-fry.

8. Garnish with sesame seeds and sliced green onions if desired.

Serving Size: This recipe serves approximately 4, offering a nutritious and satisfying meal for those on the Hyper Ketosis Diet.

Spinach and Feta Omelet with Avocado Slices

Ingredients:

- 4 large eggs
- 1 cup fresh spinach, chopped
- 1/4 cup crumbled feta cheese
- 1 ripe avocado, sliced
- 2 tablespoons butter or coconut oil
- Salt and pepper to taste
- Fresh herbs for garnish (optional, such as parsley or chives)

Instructions:

Prepare the Ingredients:

1. Crack the eggs into a bowl, add a pinch of salt and pepper, and whisk until well combined.
2. Slice the avocado and set aside for serving.

Cook the Spinach:

3. In a non-stick skillet over medium heat, add 1 tablespoon of butter or coconut oil.
4. Once melted, add the chopped spinach and sauté until wilted, about 2-3 minutes.
5. Remove the spinach from the skillet and set aside.

Make the Omelet:

6. In the same skillet, add the remaining tablespoon of butter or coconut oil.
7. Pour the whisked eggs into the skillet, swirling to cover the bottom evenly.
8. Cook the eggs for about 2 minutes, or until they start to set around the edges.

Fill the Omelet:

9. Sprinkle the cooked spinach and crumbled feta cheese over one-half of the omelet.
10. Gently fold the other half over the fillings using a spatula.

Finish Cooking:

11. Continue to cook for another 1-2 minutes until the eggs are fully set and the cheese is slightly melted.

Serve:

12. Slide the omelet onto a plate and serve with the sliced avocado on the side.
13. Garnish with fresh herbs if desired.

Serving Size: This recipe makes 2 servings, offering a nutritious and satisfying breakfast for those on the Hyper Ketosis Diet.

Grilled Chicken Salad

Ingredients:

- 2 boneless, skinless chicken breasts
- 6 cups mixed greens (such as arugula, spinach, and romaine)
- 1 red bell pepper, sliced
- 1 yellow bell pepper, sliced
- 1/4 cup olive oil
- 2 tablespoons lemon juice
- 1 teaspoon Dijon mustard
- Salt and pepper to taste
- Fresh herbs for garnish (optional, such as basil or parsley)

Instructions:

Grill the Chicken:

1. Preheat your grill or grill pan to medium-high heat.
2. Season the chicken breasts with salt and pepper.
3. Grill the chicken for 6-7 minutes on each side, or until fully cooked and the internal temperature reaches 165°F (75°C).
4. Remove from the grill and let rest for a few minutes before slicing.

Prepare the Dressing:

5. In a small bowl, whisk together the olive oil, lemon juice, and Dijon mustard.
6. Season with salt and pepper to taste.

Assemble the Salad:

7. In a large salad bowl, combine the mixed greens and sliced bell peppers.
8. Drizzle the olive oil dressing over the salad and toss to coat evenly.

Serve:

9. Divide the salad among four plates.
10. Top each plate with slices of grilled chicken.
11. Garnish with fresh herbs if desired.

Serving Size: This recipe serves approximately 4, providing a fresh and nutritious meal for those following the Hyper Ketosis Diet.

Baked Salmon with Broccoli and Cauliflower Rice

Ingredients:

- 4 salmon filets (about 6 oz each)
- 1 large head of broccoli, cut into florets
- 1 medium head of cauliflower, grated or processed into rice
- 3 tablespoons olive oil
- 2 tablespoons lemon juice
- 2 cloves garlic, minced
- Salt and pepper to taste
- Fresh dill or parsley for garnish (optional)

Instructions:

Prepare the Oven and Salmon:

1. Preheat your oven to 400°F (200°C).
2. Place the salmon filets on a baking sheet lined with parchment paper.
3. In a small bowl, mix together 2 tablespoons of olive oil, lemon juice, garlic, salt, and pepper.
4. Brush the mixture over the salmon filets.

Bake the Salmon:

5. Bake the salmon in the preheated oven for 12-15 minutes or until the fish flakes easily with a fork.

Steam the Broccoli:

6. While the salmon is baking, bring a pot of water to a boil.
7. Place the broccoli florets in a steamer basket over the boiling water.
8. Cover and steam for 5-7 minutes, or until the broccoli is tender-crisp.

Prepare the Cauliflower Rice:

9. In a large skillet, heat the remaining tablespoon of olive oil over medium heat.
10. Add the grated or processed cauliflower and sauté for 5-6 minutes until the cauliflower is tender and slightly golden.
11. Season with salt and pepper to taste.

Serve:

12. Divide the cauliflower rice among four plates.
13. Top with a salmon filet and a portion of steamed broccoli.
14. Garnish with fresh dill or parsley if desired.

Serving Size: This recipe serves 4, providing a nutritious and satisfying meal for those following the Hyper Ketosis Diet.

Conclusion

Congratulations on completing the Hyper Ketosis Diet Guide for Women! By reaching this point, you've already demonstrated a commitment to improving your health and lifestyle. This guide is designed to empower you with the knowledge and tools needed to make informed decisions about your diet and well-being.

As you continue your journey with the Hyper Ketosis diet, remember that consistency is key. This dietary approach offers a wealth of benefits, from increased energy levels and mental clarity to potential weight loss and improved metabolic health. However, like any significant lifestyle change, it can come with its challenges. It's important to be patient with yourself as you adapt to a new way of eating. Cravings and moments of doubt may arise, but with determination and the right mindset, you can overcome them.

Self-care should be an integral part of your journey. Listen to your body and understand its needs. If you feel fatigued or notice other changes, consider adjusting your diet or consulting with a healthcare professional. Remember, this is not just about losing weight or achieving a certain body image; it's about nurturing your body and mind, fostering a healthier version of yourself.

Community support can be incredibly beneficial as you navigate this diet. Engaging with others who are on a similar path can provide encouragement, tips, and recipes to keep your meals exciting and varied. Join online forums, and local groups, or even start a blog to share your experiences and learn from others. The support system you build will be invaluable not just for motivation but also for sharing practical advice.

Exploring new recipes is a fantastic way to keep your meals enjoyable and your motivation high. The sample recipes provided in this guide are just the starting point. Challenge yourself to experiment with different ingredients and cooking methods. The more you diversify your meals, the less likely you are to feel restricted. Each new dish is an opportunity to discover flavors and textures that you love, making the diet sustainable in the long term.

As you continue, celebrate every victory, no matter how small. Each day you adhere to your dietary goals is a step toward a healthier future. If you face setbacks, don't be discouraged. Use them as learning experiences to refine your approach and strengthen your resolve. Progress is rarely linear; what matters is your dedication to moving forward.

Your decision to embrace this diet is a testament to your strength and desire for a healthier lifestyle. You have the power to transform your well-being with each meal choice you make. Keep in mind the vision of who you want to become and let it drive you toward your goals. With each recipe you try and each day you commit to your plan, you're laying the foundation for long-term health and happiness.

Finally, thank you for taking the time to engage with this guide. Your dedication to understanding and implementing the Hyper Ketosis diet is commendable. As you move forward, know that you have the tools and support to succeed. Embrace the journey, enjoy the process, and remember that you are capable of achieving amazing things.

FAQs

What are the primary benefits of the Hyper Ketosis Diet for women?

The Hyper Ketosis Diet primarily enhances energy levels, sharpens mental clarity, and supports effective weight management. By focusing on a high-fat, low-carb nutritional plan, it helps the body enter a state of ketosis, where fat is used as the main energy source, leading to these beneficial outcomes.

Are there any side effects associated with the Hyper Ketosis Diet?

Some women may experience temporary side effects, such as the "keto flu," which includes symptoms like fatigue, headache, and nausea. These are generally short-lived and can be alleviated by staying hydrated, replenishing electrolytes, and consuming adequate healthy fats.

How does the Hyper Ketosis Diet differ from other ketogenic diets?

While similar to traditional ketogenic diets, the Hyper Ketosis Diet is tailored specifically for women's wellness needs, focusing more on hormonal balance and nutritional requirements unique to women. It often includes specific meal plans and recipes designed to support female health.

What should I consider before starting the Hyper Ketosis Diet?

Before beginning the diet, consider consulting with a healthcare professional, especially if you have underlying health conditions or are pregnant. It's also important to prepare for a dietary shift and ensure you have access to the right foods and resources to support your transition.

Can I follow the Hyper Ketosis Diet if I am pregnant or breastfeeding?

It's crucial to consult with a healthcare provider before starting the Hyper Ketosis Diet if you are pregnant or breastfeeding. Nutritional needs are heightened during these periods, and your doctor can help determine if this diet is appropriate for you.

What tips can help me succeed on the Hyper Ketosis Diet?

Success on the Hyper Ketosis Diet can be enhanced by planning meals ahead, maintaining hydration, tracking your macronutrient intake, and joining support groups for motivation. It's also beneficial to regularly monitor your progress to make necessary adjustments.

Are there specific foods I should prioritize or avoid on this diet?

Prioritize high-fat, low-carb foods such as avocados, nuts, seeds, oils, and fatty fish. Avoid high-carb foods like grains, sugars, and most fruits. The focus should be on whole, unprocessed foods that support the ketogenic state.

References and Helpful Links

Ld, S. S. M. R. (2023, February 23). 20 foods to eat on the keto diet. Healthline. https://www.healthline.com/nutrition/ketogenic-diet-foods

Keto for Women: 14 Tips and Recipes to help you get results | Thrive Market. (2022, March 14). Thrive Market. https://thrivemarket.com/blog/keto-for-women-tips-and-recipes-to-help-you-get-results#:~:text=In%20her%20practice%20as%20a,irregularities%2C%20and%20experience%20thyroid%20imbalances.

Brighten, J. (2024, August 25). Keto for Women: the risks, benefits, and how it impacts hormones. Dr. Jolene Brighten. https://drbrighten.com/keto-and-womens-health/

Professional, C. C. M. (2024, May 1). Ketosis. Cleveland Clinic. https://my.clevelandclinic.org/health/articles/24003-ketosis#:~:text=The%20keto%20diet%20has%20many%20benefits%2C%20but%20it%20may%20come,(%E2%80%9Cketo%E2%80%9D%20breath).

Hyper Ketosis Diet: A Complete Guide and Cookbook with . . .. (n.d.). Goodreads. https://www.goodreads.com/book/show/218412963-hyper-ketosis-diet

Amazon.com: Hyper Ketosis Diet: A comprehensive guide to delicious recipes and Cutting-Edge Ketosis Techniques for maximum fat burning For Beginners | Includes a 30-Day meal plan and shopping list: 9798336265422: A. Rojas RD, Julius: Books. (n.d.-b).

https://www.amazon.com/Hyper-Ketosis-Diet-Comprehensive-Cutting-Edge/dp/B0DDKWGFLF#:~:text=The%20Hyper%20Ketosis%20Diet%20is%20highly%20effective%20in%20stabilizing%20blood,lead%20to%20better%20overall%20health.

Fletcher, J. (2023, October 20). How to get into ketosis faster. https://www.medicalnewstoday.com/articles/324599

www.ingramcontent.com/pod-product-compliance
Lightning Source LLC
LaVergne TN
LVHW012030060526
838201LV00061B/4546